Sleep

Natural Remedies and Recipes to Sleep Better, Increase Your Health, Energy and Happiness

Contents

The trademarks that are used are without any consent, and the publication of the trademark is without permission or backing by the trademark owner. All trademarks and brands within this book are for clarifying purposes only and are the owned by the owners themselves, not affiliated with this document.

Chapter 1. The Importance of Better Sleep

What most people don't realize is that sleep is extremely important to your mental, emotional health and even your physical health. You need sleep to function properly, and it goes passed the capacity to think clearly, and it can even affect ADD, ADHD, bipolar, depression, and anxiety attacks. There are many ailments that a lack of sleep can cause and more sleep can fix, but getting sleep isn't always easy. You don't need to turn to over the counter or prescription medication because there are many natural solutions to any sleep problems that you may be experiencing, but first you have to truly understand the importance of sleep when it comes to staying healthy.

What Sleep Really Is:

Sleep is more than just a way to dream or pass the hours of night away until the sun comes back out. It's a time that your body recovers from everything that happened during the day, and it's needed for each and every one without exception. Of course, some people can deal with less sleep than others, but it's still healthy to get seven and a half to nine hours of sleep at night for a healthy adult.

Sleep is the time for brain chemicals to be restored and the body gets to rest after you've used it for hours on end. You'll be able to organize and store your memories during sleep, and a lack of sleep can cause these memories to fade away no matter how young or old you are.

Without sleep, you'll become drowsy even when you're awake, and you'll feel much less alert. Basic activities can become dangerous because your reflexes aren't sharp, and your hand eye coordination will suffer. This can make cutting vegetables all the way to driving dangerous, so sleep is needed for you to rest and think clearly. It will allow your body to react better and faster the next day, just like your mind.

All Sleep Isn't Good Sleep:

You need to also understand that just because you're getting sleep doesn't mean that you're getting good sleep. There is a difference between good sleep and just sleep, and if you are getting bad sleep, then you're most likely having your sleep cycle interrupted and the sleep is restless in comparison. Your muscles won't be relaxed, and your body will constantly be tossing and turning. This can lead to you waking up feeling more exhausted than you went to bed, and your blood circulation can even be disrupted, causing nightmares and soreness when you wake up, as well as numb limbs.

When you get good sleep, your blood circulation is fine, you don't roll more than a few times, you're restful, and your sleep is usually uninterrupted. Your muscles shouldn't be sore when you get up, and you'll be able to go through the five stages of sleep more than once. You don't go through the five stages once if you're getting good sleep because that's not enough. You should have at least two hours of dreaming, which is where you've reached the R.E.M. stage, which is one of the best ways to get a restful sleep that will help your mind to sort itself out and even process everything that you've went through during that day, emotionally, mentally and physically.

REM is where your thoughts will be sorted out and brain signals will be made sense of. It's where you're dreaming, and it'll make more connections in your brain to help you remember what happened easier, helping you to recall anything that you learned the day before. Of course, it's not just about dreams. During this your body will also begin to produce and even store proteins that help to restore and even renew your body for the upcoming day.

How to Know if You're Getting Bad Sleep:

If you're getting bad sleep, you probably already know it. Of course, that's usually if it's progressed opt the point of starting to affect your daily life. If you know the signs of bad sleep, you'll be able to recognize and correct it before it becomes a harmful cycle. You'll have a hard time staying awake during the day, including during activities such as working or driving. You will feel tire when you wake up, and you'll feel inactive and tired when watching TV or just going about you day.

You may blink more frequently, and you're more likely to yawn more often during the day. Your thoughts may feel disconnected, and daydreaming is actually a sign of not getting enough sleep. You may have a hard time with your attention span or concentration, and your memory will become faded or you'll at least have problems recalling information. You may start to take naps more often or even experience mood swings. You may have a slower reaction time than usual, and you will dream almost immediately when you fall asleep.

If you are experiencing more than one of these symptoms, you should explore the idea that even if you are getting enough sleep it may not be restful sleep, which is affecting your daytime performance, but you shouldn't worry because there are natural solutions to the problem.

Keep Away Illness:

Getting better sleep is important for more than just a better reaction time or being able to focus a little easier. It's important because it can help you to relieve any stress, anxiety, and even stave off the effects of depression, including manic depression. If you already have bipolar, you're more likely to be able to control it naturally if you are getting enough sleep. It'll help ADD and ADHD, and if you are getting enough sleep, you are more likely to stay fit because you have the energy to exercise and manage your eating, avoiding stress eating.

This can also help you to avoid obesity and even diabetes. Your blood pressure can also be affected by your sleep, and anger management becomes that much easier when you're getting the sleep that your body needs because you'll be able to rationalize events as they happen a little easier.

An Overview of Benefits:

There are benefits to getting sleep that you need, and it includes improved memory. It won't just let you remember a little easier, but it's more likely to help you focus and sharpen your memory. Your memories are known to stay sharp during old age as well, helping you to stave off Alzheimer's. Sleep is also known to help with inflammation, and inflammation is linked to heart disease, arthritis, diabetes, and even stroke. It can even lead to premature aging.

Those who sleep more are more likely to achieve their goals because the feeling of being healthier, and it can even help you in athletics due to the higher energy levels and faster reaction times that your body can produce. It'll also help you to improve your chances of success by helping you to improve your grades, due to the higher focus, sharper attention and better memory.

Sleep is known to improve your mood as well, since your body is able to process the events of the day while you're sleeping, including the stress related to it. The bottom line is, that when you get enough sleep you're more likely to be a happy, healthy and successful person.

Chapter 2. Homemade Teas to Help

You may be asking how you can improve your sleep without prescription drugs or over the counter pills, and there are many natural remedies. However, homemade teas are usually the most common way to make sure that you have something that will help you to sleep. There are many tea remedies that you can make, and some of them are extremely easy.

Sleep Tea #1 Passionflower Sedative

What most people don't know about the passionflower is that it helps you to sleep because it is actually a sedative. It's much more than a pretty flower, and it can actually knock you out. Passionflower produces a lovely taste that is enjoyed by many people, and you're able to add it into any tea leaves that you already have. This basic tea is great, and remember to add honey to sweeten. White tea is the base because it has no caffeine, but the orange is just added to add a little more flavor.

Ingredients:

1. 2 Teaspoons Passionflower Leaves
2. 2 Tablespoons White Tea Leaves
3. ½ Teaspoon Dried Orange Peel

Directions:

1. Just boil the water, and then make sure to add in the ingredients. All of the ingredients can be added in at the same time, and you will want to reduce the heat to simmer.

2. Simmer for five to ten minutes, depending on how strong you want your tea.

3. Make sure to strain out all of the herbs, including the orange peel so it shouldn't be grated.

4. Next, add sweetener if desired.

Sleep Tea #2 Basic Chamomile

Chamomile is known to relax you, including your muscles while being great to help sort your anxiety as well. This is great if you're already stressed or depressed. Of course, you'll find that adding just a little bit of lemon balm is also helpful because it'll help you to relax your muscles even more, and the scent is considered to be therapeutic. Adding a dash of cinnamon is mostly for flavor. Remember to sweeten with honey, as it promotes relaxation as well. Never add sugar to your sleepy time tea.

Ingredients:

1. 2 Teaspoons Chamomile Flowers
2. 1 Teaspoon Lemon Balm
3. ½ Teaspoon Cinnamon

Directions:

1. Boil your water, and when it comes to a boil, add in all of your ingredients.
2. Make sure to let it simmer, bringing it down from a boil and stirring occasionally. Let it simmer for six to eight minutes before taking it off.
3. Strain out the herbs, and add any honey if desired. Drink while warm.

Sleep Tea #3 Valerian Knockout

If you're having a very hard time sleeping and a basic tea won't cut it, then try a basic valerian tea. Valerian is great if you're suffering from severe sleep issues, including but not limited to insomnia.

Just remember to use valerian very carefully, as it is an herb that you can overdose on. Only take it once a day, and always tell your doctor when you plan to use it. The peppermint is added for its soothing qualities both when you drink it, as it soothes your digestive system, but the smell is also known to help sooth your nerves and stress away.

Ingredients:

1. 1 Teaspoon Valerian Herb
2. 4-6 Drops Peppermint Extract

Directions:

1. Boil your water, adding in the valerian and then stirring in the peppermint extract.

2. Reduce to a simmer, and let simmer for six to eight minutes.

3. Strain out the valerian root before adding any honey and drinking.

Sleep Tea #4 Spiced Tea

If you're looking for a tea with a little more flavor, you can add in the chamomile that is sure to help you relax your muscles and nutmeg which is known to help produce natural and better sleep. The cinnamon is added in once again for flavor, and the peppermint extract is going to make sure that the spices do not upset your stomach before bed while also giving a therapeutic effect from the smell.

Ingredients:

1. 2 Teaspoons Chamomile Flowers

2. 2 Nutmegs, Quartered or Grated

3. ½ Cinnamon Stick

4. 4-6 Drops Peppermint Extract

Directions:

1. Boil your water, adding in all of your ingredients. If you don't have cinnamon sticks, you can use grated cinnamon as well.
2. Bring it down to a simmer, letting it simmer for about five to ten minutes.
3. Add in honey as desired after straining, and drink while warm.

Sleep Tea #5 Infused Green Tea

Green tea may have a little caffeine, but it also is known to help with natural sleep, and it can help relieve the stress that is keeping you up. Of course, in this tea it's infused with saffron, which is also known to help you to get to sleep naturally due to its mild sedative properties. Dried strawberries are added to help make the tea a little more flavorful, but you can always add any dried fruit that you want. Most people will use dried orange peel, since it's easy to get ahold of.

Ingredients:

1. 2 Teaspoons Green Tea Leaves
2. 1 Teaspoon Saffron, Dried
3. 2 Teaspoons Dried Strawberries

Directions:

1. It doesn't have to be whole dried strawberries, and it's actually recommended that it is. Add in all ingredients when you bring the water to a boil, and then reduce it to a simmer.
2. Let it simmer for five to ten minutes to infuse throughout the water.
3. Strain out everything, and then add honey if desired to drink while warm.

Sleep Tea #6 A Mild Sleep Aid

If you're looking for something a little milder to help, then this is a relaxing tea that will help you to break the cycle of bad sleep. Take it about thirty minutes before bed, and remember to only sweeten with honey, as it'll also help you to relax your muscles. The lavender also has aromatherapy qualities, which help you to relax and relive your stress, but when taken internally it'll act as a mild sedative, much like saffron. Chamomile is also a way to help relieve stress and anxiety, helping you to relax your muscles. Peppermint is going to relax any digestive issues, and help you to sleep through its aromatherapy properties as well.

Ingredients:

1. 2 Teaspoons Lavender, Dried

2. 1 ½ Teaspoon Chamomile Flowers, Dried

3. 5-7 Drops Peppermint Extract

Directions:

1. Boil your water, adding in all ingredients as you reduce it to a simmer. You even need to stir in your peppermint extract.
2. Let it finish simmering for eight to ten minutes, and then strain out all flowers.
3. Sweeten and drink while it's still warm. Remember that a teaspoon of peppermint leaves can be used if you do not have peppermint extract.

Sleep Tea #8 Lemon Balm Delight

If you're looking for a sleep tea that is going to relax your muscles and your mind so that you get the sleep you need, then try this one. Of course, you'll find that honey helps with sleep as well, and the ginger is going to help with any aches and pains that may be keeping you up. The holy basil will help you to relieve your stress and get to sleep faster as well.

Ingredients:

1. 1 Teaspoon Holy Basil, Dried
2. ½ Teaspoon Powdered Ginger
3. 2 Teaspoons Honey, Raw
4. 2 Tablespoons Lemon Balm

Directions:

1. Make sure to boil water, steeping the herbs in it before you turn it to simmer. Let it simmer for eight to ten minutes on low.
2. Then, strain out all the herbs, making sure to add honey. Add more honey if you need it. Some people add a dash of

cinnamon for flavor and the added benefits.

Keep In Mind:

Always keep in mind that if an ingredient is added just for flavor, then you don't need it if you don't want it. You can also put in any other dried fruit in its place, or even peppermint extract. Always sweeten with honey, and it's best to buy raw, organic or local honey because it has no added sugar which will keep you up.

It'll also have more benefits, including the benefit to relax you a little more. Of course, if you only have valerian, passionflower, green tea, lavender, chamomile, lemon balm, or peppermint leaves, you can use boiled water and turn these single herbs into a tea as well. Of course, it won't be as strong as the tea mixes

above as it's only a single ingredient made into
a tea.

Chapter 3. Some Tea Baths That Work

You may be asking what a tea bath is, but it's actually herbs that you put into a hot bath, like you would a tea, and then you soak in them. This is another way to use natural herbs to cure your sleep problem, and it really works. Hot baths work on their own because it raises your body temperature slightly, and when you get out it mimics your body temperature dropping, just as it does when your body prepared for sleep. This will help you to get natural sleep, but with herbs mixed in, the process is perfected to help you eliminate anything holding you back from restful and long sleep that will help you recover from your day.

Tea Bath #1 A Rosy Feeling

This is a bath that works mostly because of its aromatherapy benefits, but it works. It helps to relax your muscles, and it'll help you to relive your stress. You'll need essential oils, including rose and peppermint. Rose is relaxing, and peppermint helps to make you feel awake and a little more sensitive. It may seem counterproductive, but it's a great way to get rid of your stress. You'll also want dried lavender flower and rose petals, which will soak into the hot water to help you sleep as well.

Ingredients:

1. 7-10 Drops Rose Oil
2. 1 Handful Rose Petals
3. 2 Teaspoons Lavender, Dried
4. 2-5 Drops Peppermint Oil

Directions:

1. Just heat your bath up, and mix everything in. relax for at least twenty to thirty minutes to get the full effects of a tea bath.

Tea Bath #2 The Calming Bath

If you're looking for something to calm your nerves because your stress and anxiety is going to keep you up that night, then try this bath. The chamomile is extremely relaxing, and it's common to use in a tea bath. Of course, helpful essential oils are still needed, including lavender oil and a little more rose oil. You'll be able to enjoy your bath, and the chamomile is known to help you relax any sore muscles you may have.

Ingredients:

1. 4 Tablespoons Chamomile Flowers, Dried

2. 4-6 Drops Rose Oil

3. 5-8 Drops Lavender Oil

Directions:

1. Make sure to either brew the chamomile
    flowers first or put them in the hot water
    while the tub is filling up to give them
    more time to steep.
2. Then add in your essential oils, and relax
    for twenty to thirty minutes.

Tea Bath #3 Spiced Soak

Ginger is great for your sore muscles, which is
commonly what's keeping you up at night. If
you find that this tea bath is not strong enough,
just add more ginger and brew the tea before
adding it into the water instead of trying to do
so in the tub. This is often a more potent form
of any tea bath, including any spice soaks. It
can also help if you're sick, including with a

runny nose, cough, cold or even the flu. The milk is just great for your skin, and it'll help to relax you and therefore your muscles as well.

Ingredients:

1. 1 Medium Piece Ginger
2. 1 Cup Milk

Directions:

1. Start by peeling and slicing your ginger.
2. Add the sliced ginger into the hot water, making sure to mix thoroughly.
3. Then, you can add your milk to the mixture. Try to make sure it's at least room temperature before you put it in so you don't lower the temperature of the overall bath.

Tea Bath #4 Sage Bath

If you're looking for something that's going to relax you to sleep and help get rid of oily skin or acne, then sage baths are probably for you. It's a dried herb that you usually already have in your kitchen cabinet, and with a few extra essential oils, you're sure to be happy. Add just a few drops of peppermint for its aromatherapy, and a few drops rose also helps for the same reason.

Ingredients:

1. ¼ Cup Dried Sage
2. 4-5 Drops Peppermint Oil
3. 5-8 Drops Rose Oil

Directions:

1. Mix in the dried herbs to the bath first.
2. Once the sage is mixed into the hot water, add in the essential oils.

Bath Tea #5 Salt Bath

Epsom salt is great at relaxing you and your muscles. It'll help with stress, and when added with natural herbs the effects are amazing. Lavender is known to be a great aid for sleep and relaxation, and dried lavender works just as well as any lavender essential oil. Some people even say that it works better. What some people don't know is that Epsom salt is also a great way to boost your immune system.

Ingredients:

1. 1 Cup Epsom Salts
2. ½ Cup Dried Lavender

Directions:

1. Mix in the Epsom salts and lavender at the same time, making sure that you have hot water.

Bath Tea #6 Chamomile & Milk

If you're looking for one that's sure to knock you out, try adding zero stimulants with this chamomile and milk bath. Not only is it good for your sleep schedule, but it's also good for your skin. The milk makes you feel relaxed, and it makes your skin soft and rejuvenated. The chamomile is sure to release tension in your muscles and remove anxiety as well. When added with honey to make your skin extra soft, including with anti-aging properties, and lavender oil to help you relieve any leftover stress, this tea bath is great for right before bed.

Ingredients:

1. ¾ Cup Warm Milk
2. ½ Cup Chamomile Flowers, Dried
3. 5-8 Drops Lavender Oil
4. 3 Tablespoons Raw Honey

Directions:

1. Add in the warm milk, lavender oil, and honey first with the warm water.
2. Add in and stir in dried chamomile.

Bath Tea #7 Earthy Delight

If you're looking for something that doesn't smell too much like flowers but will still do the trick to make it where you sleep better, then this is the bath tea for you. It's great at making sure you relax your muscles, ease stress, and that no pain is keeping you up. Add in the Epsom salts, and you're sure to fall asleep quickly afterwards. Rosemary is a great anti-inflammatory, and it's good for aromatherapy for stress as well. Ginger is sure to help you relax your muscles as well, and the dried lavender does the sleepy time trick.

Ingredients:

1. 1 Piece Ginger
2. ¼ Cup Dried Rosemary
3. ¼ Cup Dried Lavender
4. ½ Cup Epsom Salts

1. Everything can be added to this tea bath together, and then you can soak in it for as long as you need to.

Chapter 4. Basic Foods to Use & Add In

There are many foods that you can add to your diet that will help you to sleep as well, but you can't expect results to be immediate. Often, if you are using food to help you sleep, then you'll find that there are more long term results with changing your diet and incorporating these foods in.

Short term effects can be felt by some people, but they're often not nearly as prominent as the long term benefits. To use foods to help with your sleep, you don't have to drastically change your diet. Just try to add as many of these foods into your diet as possible, so that you are promoting better sleep throughout your day.

Almonds:

Magnesium rich food is good for quality sleep because magnesium is a mineral that you need for quality sleep. If your magnesium levels are too low, you're much more likely to wake up periodically through the night. By eating almonds a few times a week, you're more likely to get restful sleep when you do end up falling asleep. You don't even have to change your sleep schedule.

Lettuce:

Eating a salad with dinner is healthier in more ways than once, and that's because lettuce contains lactucarium. This has sedative properties, and it actually affects your brain in a similar fashion to opium, but to a much lesser extent. You can actually make a tea from lettuce leaves by taking three to five large leaves, adding them into a cup of water for fifteen minutes. Then you just add mint and heat it up to sip at before bed. Of course, eating a salad is also known to work pretty well.

Tuna:

Everyone knows that tuna is brain food, but it's actually sleep food as well. It has needed vitamin B6, which your body needs to be able to properly produce both serotonin and melatonin. This is needed for sleep, and a deficiency in B6 can lead to bad sleep and a bad sleep cycle overall. Of course, for the same reason you could add in garlic or even pistachios into your diet to help you out.

White Rice:

Not every rice is helpful for your sleep, but white rice is. It has a high glycemic index, meaning it'll help you to fall asleep much faster.

Of course, jasmine rice is known to bring sleep the fastest. If you eat other rice types, it's sure to help some, but not in the same way, and not quickly. Try not to eat it too early in the day, but adding it into your dinners will produce both short term and long term effects.

Honey:

This is great if you're already using teas to help you fall asleep and get better sleep, but it's good to use honey on its own. You can use it by baking with it, but you won't get the same effects as if you ate the honey raw. It's a natural sugar, and it will raise your insulin levels slightly, allowing tryptophans to enter the brain. This is what results in helping you to sleep.

Kale:

If you don't want to add more lettuce in your diet, trying adding kale if you want better sleep. It has tons of calcium, and calcium is needed to help tryptophans to make melatonin. If you can't stand kale's bitter taste, try spinach, including baby spinach, or even mustard greens to get the calcium you need because milk won't cut it.

Cherry Juice:

Tart cherry juice is best, and try to make sure it isn't a cherry juice cocktail. It's a great sleep aide because its melatonin rich, and it'll help you to sleep quickly. It helps if you're having mild sleeping issues, but over time it can actually even help relieve the severity of insomnia. However, you need to drink it twice daily for the best results.

Yogurt:

Greek yogurt is actually best, and try to find yogurt that is unsweetened or sweetened with honey if you want strong, healthy results. This is because it'll boost the amount of calcium that you're getting, which will help you to fall asleep. If you are calcium deficient, you are prone to having a harder time falling asleep, reducing your quality and quantity of sleep over time.

Barley:

If you don't like barley, other whole grains like bulgur work as well. However, it's because they are rich in magnesium, and it'll help you to stay asleep. If you don't have enough, you're going to be waking up more often. Try to incorporate them into at least one daily meal so that your magnesium levels don't dip too low.

Bananas:

Bananas are harder to work into your daily diet, but they're still good for sleep because they are rich in B6, helping you to produce the needed melatonin. It's a sleep inducing hormone that will help you to enrich your quality of sleep, but over time it will help with your quantity of sleep as well.

Oatmeal:

Oatmeal is a great breakfast, but it's also great if you want to make sure that your blood sugars are raised naturally. Once your blood sugars are raised, you're going to feel sleepier, and eating oats also helps by raising your melatonin levels, which will relax your body so that you can get to sleep. Oatmeal is great right before bed, and you can actually use oatmeal as your dinner, especially if you aren't feeling too well.

Dark Chocolate:

If you're looking for the perfect nighttime snack, try eating dark chocolate. Milk chocolate is more of a stimulant, but if you eat dark chocolate then you're getting the needed serotonin which will relax both your mind and body. Just remember that the higher the percentage of cocoa the better the dark chocolate is.

Turkey:

Everyone knows that you get sleepy after Thanksgiving dinner, but it actually does have tryptophan in it. This will help you gain both serotonin and melatonin once it's metabolized, causing your body to want to doze off. There are still many people that argue that it isn't the turkey that makes you sleepy but the amount you eat, but eating it more regularly is going to help you to sleep a little more soundly.

Some Foods to Avoid:

Just like there are foods that can help you with sleep, there are also many foods to avoid if you don't want to get bad sleep. Spicy foods are one of them. Spicy foods are sure to upset your stomach and keep you up for the majority of the night. Caffeinated drinks are also something you should avoid before sleep, including caffeinated food such as milk chocolate. The stimulant in it will keep you up. This includes ginseng tea. It's a great herbal tea, and it's very healthy, but when you're trying to sleep it's a proven stimulant that is more likely to just keep you up. Alcohol also isn't good if you're looking for quality sleep because it'll actually keep your body from reaching deep stages of sleep.

Chapter 5. Supplements for a Proper Solution

There are many natural supplements that you can still take to help you sleep, and it works even better if you're paring it with herbal teas or food that is going to help you sleep. Of course, a good diet and exercise also contribute to quality and quantity sleep, even if the supplements below are going to help.

Valerian:

This is an herb that is often recommended to help you get to sleep faster, and you can get it in its supplement form to help you get to sleep fast. It has sedative properties, which is known to help increase gamma-aminobutyric acid, which helps the brain from transmitting nerve impulses. It is often great when combined with hops, but taking a valerian supplement on its own is a great natural sleep solution.

Melatonin:

If you're having a hard time falling asleep at night, then you probably need more melatonin, and that's because it will help with an abnormal sleep and wake cycle. This is great for parents who have a young child because it'll help you to get to sleep a little faster each time you get woken up. It's a hormone that is released throughout the day, helping you to stay alert when you need to and rest when you need to.

Holy Basil:

If you're experiencing stress, and that's the reason for your lack of sleep or your bad quality of sleep, then you might want to try a holy basil supplement. It helps to disrupt the rhythm of cortisol, which will spike from six to eight in the morning for most people, but with stress, it'll make your cortisol spike differently. Holy basil helps to moderate it, which helps you to calm down to sleep through the night during a normal sleep schedule. It even helps with anxiety and mild depression. One to two capsules are usually taken in the early evening for the best results.

5-HTP:

Also known as F-hydroxytrptophane, 5-HTP, is great if you're struggling with depression. This is a mood boosting supplement that will help you to get a little more sleep despite any depression or bad mood. Many people who are having a hard time sleeping will actually be suffering from sleep depression, but this supplements is what melatonin is made from that will then convert to serotonin, helping you to feel better. It's equally beneficial for your mood as it is for your sleep.

Magnesium:

Many people don't have enough magnesium in their system, and it always works best if you're taking it with calcium as well. Magnesium is important to the body because it'll help you to aid in sleep by relaxing your muscles and it can even calm your nerves. Sadly, most people are actually deficient in magnesium, so it's in many sleep supplement formulas.

B-Vitamins:

There are many B-vitamins that are important to your sleep schedule because they help your tryptophan to convert into niacin and serotonin. This helps to regulate sleep, and it helps to increase REM. REM is extremely important when it comes to getting better quality of sleep.

Vitamin D:

Many people are also actually low in their vitamin D, which can cause you to be drowsy during the day. It can help you to improve your overall well-being if you fix any vitamin D deficiency in your body, and this includes helping to promote better sleep.

Theanine:

This is another amino acid which is often found in green tea, and it helps to trigger the brain to release gamma-aminobutyric acid, and it helps you to calm your nerves. It helps you to reduce anxiety, and it this is one of the main reasons it'll help you to get to sleep quickly.

Multi-Vitamin:

Most people underestimate what a multi-vitamin can actually do for you. Sadly, most people aren't actually getting enough vitamins from their meals because they aren't easting as healthy as they should. This is one of the main reasons that it'll help you to get to sleep. A lack of nutrients will keep you up at night because you aren't producing the chemicals you need for sleep.

Keep in Mind:

When you add a supplement, you need to follow the directions on the bottle. You will also want to tell your doctor before you start taking a supplement if you are on any over the counter or prescription medication, as there are certain supplements that will interact with certain medications. Your doctor will be able to tell you if you're taking the right supplement to go with your medications as well as to help you if you have a deficiency. If you worry about having a deficiency, your doctor can causally check with a simple blood test. Always keep in mind that

stacking supplements with good sleep
producing habits is always best as well.

Chapter 6. More Herbal Remedies to Try

If you're still having a hard time sleeping, some people need other remedies besides just tea, and you'll find that there are many natural remedies out there that can help. You are using the same thing that you would in tea for most of the time, but there are different ways to take it. You don't have to drink a tea if you don't want to.

Remedy #1 Sleep Well Salve

You can actually use a salve to help you sleep better, and this way you can experience the benefits of an herbal remedy without having to drink anything at all. This salve is known to help because it helps you to calm your nerves and fight any stress that is keeping you up. It has the added benefits of making your hands and feet smooth. You can use it for yourself, but it also works as a great gift.

Ingredients:

1. 1 Cup Organic Coconut Oil
2. 1 Cup Olive Oil
3. 4 Tablespoons Beeswax, Grated
4. 8-10 Drops Cedar Wood Essential Oil
5. 8-10 Drops Orange Essential Oil
6. 8-10 Drops Cinnamon Essential Oil
7. 8-10 Drops Peppermint Essential Oil

Directions:

1. Make sure to heat up your olive oil, beeswax, and coconut oil. Heat it up over a double boiler, and then stir it.
2. Add in all of your essential oil, continuing to stir.

3. Pour into a sealed glass container, and
   let it cool.

Remedy #2 A Gummy Solution

If you love gummies, you can always use these magnesium gummies to help you get to sleep quickly. It'll work instead of taking a supplement, and it actually tastes pretty good.

Ingredients:

1. ¾ Cup Juice of Your Choice, Organic
2. 3 Tablespoons Gelatin Powder
3. 5 Tablespoons Magnesium Citrate Powder
4. 1 Tablespoon Honey
5. 1/8 Teaspoon Sea Salt, Fine

Directions:

1. Your juice should be refrigerated, and then you can pour it into a medium-large mixing bowl, and then whisk the magnesium powder in until it foams up. It is usually best to whisk a single tablespoon at a time, and then continue to whisk until the foam goes down.

2. Take a small saucepan, and add in the juice mixture. Put the gelatin powder over it, but don't add heat yet. The gelatin powder needs to be left so that it can "bloom", which is where the gelatin powder begins to absorb the liquid. You need to give it a few minutes, or you will have a gritty gummy.

3. Turn the burner on, and don't put it above low-medium heat. It should liquefy, and then you can add in your honey and salt.

4. Whisk it together, but not too much or it'll foam up.

5. Pour it into a silicone mold and let sit.

6. Refrigerate until its set.

Remedy #3 Another Helpful Salve

This is a salve that uses chamomile which will actually help to alleviate any aches and pains that you might having issues with. It will also soothe any inflammation. Lemon balm is also used to help with any anxiety that you may be experiencing, including depression. Its' even known to have small sedatives, and lavender will help to promote sleep by easing stress.

Ingredients:

1. ¼ cup Lemon Balm, Dried

2. ¼ Cup Chamomile Flowers, Dried

3. 8-10 Lavender Essential Oil

4. 1 Teaspoon Vitamin E Oil

5. 1 ½ Cup Organic Coconut Oil

6. 2 Tablespoons Beeswax, Grated

Directions:

1. Your oven needs to be turned to 200 degrees, and then you need to turn it off once it's heated up.

2. Put in the coconut oil and herbs together into a pan. Put it in the heated oven, and let them steep for three hours.

3. Take the herbs out, and strain the now infused oil. The herbs can be tossed out once you're strained them, but keep the oil.

4. Clean out the pain, and then pour the oil back into it. Place it into a skillet on low heat, and then put in the beeswax. Let it melt, adding in the essential oil. Then, add in the vitamin E oil.

5. Make sure to mix properly, and then
    pour your balm into a jar, letting it dry.

Remedy #4 A Cinnamon Drink

You may not want a tea, but actually cinnamon can help you as well. There are many benefits of cinnamon milk, and insomnia is one of them. It also has a wonderful taste that is sure to help you feel a little better before you get to sleep. It helps to increase circulation throughout your body, which will help you to sleep better overall.

Ingredients:

1. 1 Cup Whole Milk
2. 1 Small Cinnamon Stick
3. 2 Teaspoons Honey
4. 4-5 Drops Vanilla Extract

Directions:

1. Start by heating the milk in a pan, and place the small cinnamon stick in it as well.

2. Remove it from the heat, and then add in the vanilla as well as the honey. Remember that raw honey is usually best because it has more health benefits.

3. Take out the cinnamon stick, and drink before bed.

Remedy #5 Lavender Lotion

Lotion is similar to a salve, but it does usually have less ingredients, just like this natural remedy lotion. It's easy to make, and it works pretty well. It's not as potent as some herbal remedies, but it'll help to make sure that you can relax enough to sleep, including relaxing your muscles. Remember that you should never add too much peppermint, or it could wake you up. Do not vary the amount.

Ingredients:

1. 4 Ounces Coconut Oil
2. ¾ Ounce Beeswax, Grated
3. 8-12 Drops Lavender Essential Oil
4. 2-3 Drops Peppermint Essential Oil

Directions:

1. In a double boiler, heat up the coconut oil and beeswax. Make sure to mix it together well over low to medium heat.
2. Take it off the double boiler, pouring into a glass bowl, letting it cool slightly. Whisk until fluffy, adding in essential oils as you go.
3. Spoon into glass jars when cool.

Chapter 7. Sleepy Time Smoothies to Drink

If you're still looking for a sleep remedy, you'll find that there are smoothie drinks in there that can help you as well. Smoothies are everyone's favorite, or at least for most people, but it's actually able to help you sleep if you're drinking them regularly with the right ingredients in them. These recipes are sure to taste great and help you improve your quality and quantity of sleep in a natural manner.

Smoothie #1 A Cherry Blast

Remember that tart cherry juice is actually great for helping to promote sleep. It'll help you with melatonin, and the soy milk is high in tryptophan, which is sleep-inducing. The bananas are high in magnesium which will help you to calm down, and honey is going to help with the release of melatonin as nutmeg helps to relax your muscles.

Ingredients:

1. ¾ Cup Frozen Cherry Juice
2. ¼ Cup Sliced Bananas
3. ½ Cup Cold Soy Milk
4. 2 Tablespoons Honey
5. ½ Teaspoon Nutmeg, Grated

Directions:

1. Make sure that all of your ingredients are cold, and then blend until smooth.
2. You can add in more cherry juice if desired, and ice can be added to help thicken.

Smoothie #2 Watermelon Delight

If you're looking for something that doesn't taste as tart but will help you sleep, try out this smoothie recipe. It's not as thick as other smoothies, but it's just as tasty. It'll help you to increase melatonin, and it'll even help you to relax your muscles a little bit. Honey and chamomile help you to relax and sleep as well.

Ingredients:

1. 1 Cup Frozen Cherry Juice
2. ½ Cup Watermelon, Frozen
3. ½ Cup Chamomile Tea, Frozen
4. 2 Tablespoons Honey

Directions:

1. Add all ingredients together. Make your chamomile tea in advance, making sure to freeze it. You can leave it unsweetened since you're adding honey later.

Smoothie #3 A Dreamy Blend

If you're looking for something that is blended thoroughly, and more than just a few ingredients. You'll find that this is a great smoothie for you. Honey is great for sleep, and nutmeg is going to help with any of your aches and pains. The vanilla is for flavoring, and the almonds will help with sleep as well. The cherries will help with melatonin, and the milk with calcium. The bananas are great in magnesium and potassium, which is what your body needs.

Ingredients:

1. 2 Teaspoons Honey, Raw
2. ½ Teaspoon Vanilla Extract
3. ¼ Teaspoon Nutmeg, Grated
4. ½ Cup Frozen Cherry Juice
5. 1 Sliced Banana
6. ¼ Cup Baby Spinach
7. ¼-1/2 Cup Almond Milk

Directions:

1. Add the almond milk and spinach first, blending so that it won't be stringy. Make sure it's blended properly.
2. Add in all other ingredients, and then blend thoroughly.

Smoothie #4 A Green Blend

If you're looking for more of a green smoothie that'll help you sleep, then this is a great recipe. The celery juice has a calming effect on your nervous system, which will help you to relax.

However, it also has magnesium which will promote relaxation as well. Watercress as well as romaine are both high in calcium, which will help you to relax. The lemon and orange are also used because they help to enhance your REM cycle in your sleep, which will calm anxiety and give you better quality sleep.

Ingredients:

1. 2 Oranges, Large & Peeled
2. 1 Small Lemon, Peeled
3. ½ Cup Ice
4. ½ Bunch Watercress
5. 6-8 Stalks Celery
6. ½ Cup Shredded Romaine Lettuce

Directions:

1. All ingredients need to be blended on high together. Do not add the ice until everything else is blended.

Smoothie #5 Green Tea Delight

Green tea can be a stimulant if you're using too much, but this is a great smoothie recipe if you're looking for something that is going to help you sleep while still getting your green tea fix. The theanine is a sleep supplement found in green tea that is going to help. The banana, as stated before, is going to help because of its magnesium content. The kale is high in calcium to help you relax your body.

Ingredients:

1. 1 Cup Frozen Green Tea
2. 2 Tablespoons Honey
3. ½ Cup Ice
4. ½ Cup Shredded Kale
5. 1 Large Banana, Sliced & Frozen

Directions:

1. Add in your green tea and kale first. Make sure to blend until smooth.
2. Add in all other ingredients until smooth. Add more ice if necessary to make it thicker.

Smoothie #6 A Passion for Sleep

This is a very fruity smoothie that is going to help you get to sleep. Passion fruit is the main ingredient, and it's known to help you with anxiety and stress, which will help you relax and get to sleep, including a deeper sleep. Spinach is high in calcium, and the taste is going to be covered up by the passion fruit. Milk is also high in calcium, which will help, and honey helps to promote the release of melatonin.

Ingredients:

1. ½ Cup Chopped Passion Fruit
2. 2 Tablespoons Honey
3. ½ cup Milk, Frozen
4. ½ Cup baby Spinach

Directions:

1. Add the passion fruit and spinach together first, blending until smooth.
2. Then, add in the honey and milk. Add more milk if necessary to thicken. Blend until smooth, and then drink.

Smoothie #7 Almond Butter Smoothie

Remember that almonds are great if you're having issues sleeping, and it's because they have both magnesium and calcium. You'll find that milk has more calcium, and bananas go great with this smoothie as well, giving you yet more magnesium. It can even help you to take cramps away by making sure that you are getting enough potassium in your diet.

Ingredients:

1. 5 Tablespoons Almond Butter
2. ½ Cup Frozen Whole Milk
3. 2 Bananas, Sliced & Frozen

Directions:

1. With this smoothie recipe you are able to blend everything together, and then drink it when smooth. If you really want to sweeten it, remember to add honey and not sugar. Sugar is more prone to keep you up at night.

Smoothie #8 Lemon Balm Smoothie

If you're looking for something that is going to help make sure that you have everything you need to sleep, then this lemon balm does the trick. It helps you to make sure that you get to sleep because of lemon balm's relaxing effects, and spinach helps because of its calcium. The apple is mostly for flavor, and the cucumber is just for hydration purposes.

Ingredients:

1. 1 Handful Fresh Lemon balm
2. ¼ Cup Baby Spinach
3. 1 Small Green Apple, Peeled & Cored
4. 1 Small Cucumber, Peeled
5. ½ Cup Ice

Directions:

1. Make sure to blend everything together until smooth. For a creamier texture, many people will add a half a cup of vanilla flavored Greek Yogurt.

Smoothie #9 Cherry Slush

If you're looking for more of a cherry drink that has a sweet but thick kick to it, then this is the smoothie recipe for you. Cherries are one of the best fruits to help you sleep, and the passion fruit works as a sedative as well. Of course, the milk and Greek yogurt helps to make sure you're getting the calcium you need to sleep properly. The honey helps as well, as well as being a natural sweetener.

Ingredients:

1. ½ Cup Vanilla Greek Yogurt
2. ½ Cup Frozen Cherry Juice
3. ¼ Cup Frozen Passion Fruit
4. ½ Cup Whole Milk, Frozen
5. 2 Teaspoons Raw Honey

Directions:

1. Make sure to mix everything together, and you can use fresh cherries if they are pitted as well. Frozen cherries are going to produce a thicker smoothie.

Chapter 8. Habits to Stack for Better Sleep

If you're looking for something that will help make everything a little better, then you'll find that these habits help. You can stack these habits with any other natural remedy for sleep that's found in this book. Use as many of these tricks as possible, and stack the habits to get the most out of it.

A Bedtime:

A bedtime usually works best if you're trying to get better sleep. It won't necessarily help you get more sleep unless you're making it at a time that allows you the needed hours before you have to get up. If you go to bed at the same time every night, then you're going to feel tired around that time of night as your body gets used to it. That means you are much less likely to toss and turn. It's tempting to break the routine on weekends, but try to do so as little as possible if you want the most out of this habit. If you're trying to make a drastic change, try to do it in fifteen minute increments until you're going to bed when you want to. This will prove to have the best results.

Don't Nap:

Napping is fine if you're sick, but often you really shouldn't nap during the day, especially after dinner because of drowsiness. If you're napped already, you're much less likely to be sleepy enough to go to bed when you should. If you are having a hard time staying awake, try to do something that is mildly stimulating, but don't use a stimulant like coffee or any caffeinated food or beverage. Otherwise, it's counterproductive and will probably stay in your system long enough to disrupt your sleep later on. There is an exception to the rule. You should nap only when you are trying to make up for sleep that you're losing. Instead of sleeping late in the morning because you can't get to sleep that night, sleep for a little during the day, but set an alarm so that you don't over sleep.

Don't Drink Too Much:

Don't drink too much before bed. This is including but not limited to alcohol. Drinking too much will cause you to need to go to the bathroom too much, which disrupt your sleep cycle. It'll keep you up, and often because of the light you'll have a hard time even getting back to sleep in the first place. This can keep you from entering the deeper stages of sleep, which will decrease the quality of sleep you're experiencing and leave you tired during the day even if you got enough hours.

Keep The Temperature Cool:

You need to make sure the temperature is right if you're making sure that you get enough sleep and the quality of sleep that you need. You need to make sure that the temperature isn't too cool or too hot if you're trying to sleep. It's usually best to have the temperature between sixty and sixty-seven degrees. Of course, some people need it a little warmer or cooler.

Take an Hour First:

You need to take an hour of relaxation before you go to bed. Going to bed too wound up will make it where you have a hard time sleeping. You need to dim the lights, and turn off all of your devices, and this includes laptops, phones and your TV. You need to have a quiet hour without bright lights, and reading with a reading lamp is actually recommended. However, there are other activities that you can do as well.

A Hot Bath:

Even if you aren't going to use tea baths, you might want to try a hot bath before bed if you want to get to sleep faster. A bath is going to raise your temperature, which is need for it to drop to make your body get ready for sleep. You don't need anything in your bath besides hot water, but using a tea bath will help a little more. It will also help to increase your quality of sleep, and when paired with the right schedule and the proper temperature for your room, you'll find that you sleep like a baby.

Sunlight During the Day:

Remember to get sunlight during the day. It'll help you to stay awake if you do so during the morning, but it'll also help with your production of vitamin D, which is going to keep you healthier and on the proper sleep schedule. It's best to aim for a full fifteen minutes of sun in the morning, and then try to be out in the sun for at least an hour. If you choose to get that hour all at once, then you're going to want to make sure you put on sunblock though to ensure that your skin isn't damaged.

Replace Pillows:

You're going to want to replace your pillows regularly, and that's because dust mites will actually build up in your pillow. These critters are relatively harmless except for that many people can cause you to have an allergic reaction. This can cause you to have issues sleeping because of a stuffy nose, swollen eyes, sore throat or any other allergic symptoms. Of course, it's best to replace them every few months. Many people will do so every three months, but if you're sensitive to dust mites, you may need to do so more often. Some people can get away with replacing their pillows every six months.

A Hot Drink:

Even if you aren't drinking tea or hot milk, you are going to want a hot non-caffeinated drink. The warmth of the drink is meant to relax you, and you should always choose one that's actually good on your digestive system. You don't want anything to upset your system before you go to bed. It's important to combat heart burn or acid reflux if you are prone to it.

Don't Exercise Before Bed:

Exercise is great if you're trying to make sure that you're getting tired enough and producing the chemicals you need for sleep. Of course, if you're still having a hard time sleeping, make sure that you aren't getting exercise too close to bed. This means that you'll have too much adrenaline in your system, and adrenaline is too much of a stimulant. It'll keep you awake, and even if you do get to sleep, you'll toss and turn too much to actually get the quality sleep you need.

Stack Them:

Stack all of your habits together to make sure that you get the best benefits. Even though each and every habit will actually work on its own, it won't help as much as if you were using all of them. You can stack all of these habits together, and it won't hurt you. There is no negative side effect for using these habits with one another.

Chapter 9. Bonus Tips to Help You Out

Now you know various ways to help you get to sleep from supplements to smoothies to salves, and yet there are still many tips that you can use to make sure you're getting the quality and quantity of sleep you want naturally. You never have to turn to prescription or over the counter drugs.

Wake Up at the Same Time:

Even if you're going to bed at the same time, you may not have an alarm set for the morning. However, waking up at the same time every day is going to help you to feel more rested. It'll get your body used to the schedule, and it'll make you feel less fatigued during the day. What most people don't know is that getting too much sleep can actually be detrimental to your health.

Make the Right Environment:

People think that all you need to sleep is a bed, but that isn't true. You need to have the right environment to sleep. Try to eliminate all noise and light from your bedroom. Using a blackout curtain is usually best, as it'll keep the sun from shining into the room, causing you to wake up. You can also use ear plugs or a soothing sound machine to help make sure that all noise is blocked out, especially if you're sleeping during the day. Turn your phone off, and even try to sleep with a sleep mask. Any of these distractions will interrupt your sleep cycle, and it will cause your quality to go down even if you can get back to sleep immediately so that it doesn't affect the quantity of your sleep.

Separate Blankets:

If you're sharing a bed, it's usually best to have separate blankets. It's important that the temperature stays comfortable for you when you're sleeping, or it'll disrupt your sleep cycle. Even if your partner sweats while you shiver, it can cause you to have issues sleeping. Some people even need separate beds, such as twin beds put together. You can still use a full or queen size mattress, but having a bed that fits you and keeps you at the right temperature is important. At the very least, separate blankets are needed. Make sure that you have a blanket that fits you and your room's temperature, and having more than one for different seasons and weather is usually best. You should at least have a thick and thin blanket to help you get comfortable no matter the temperature in the room.

Work Through Your Stress:

Before you go to bed, you need to make sure you work through any stress that is keeping you up. Stress, anxiety, and depression is extremely important to make sure that it doesn't keep you up. There are specific herbal teas that will help you with any anxiety or stress, but there are also other natural ways to handle any stress. One of the simplest ways is to make sure that you write out anything that's bugging you. If you write out your problems, it helps you to put them into the perspective that you need to look at the bad things that happen in life. A new perspective is always best when making sure that you can handle anxiety and stress.

Meditation and yoga is also a way that you can help to make sure that your anxiety and stress melt away before you crawl under the covers. Meditation will help you to put everything out of your mind or handle the bad in a more positive manner. Even if you just do basic breathing exercises, then you'll find out that meditating for ten to fifteen minutes before bed will help. Yoga during the day, but not too close to bedtime, will help you to keep your stress down as well.

Remember:

No matter what, make sure that you stack your habits to get the best result. You can also stack these tips and remedies. You can use smoothies, salves, and teas together, for example, in the same day to help make sure that you get restful sleep and can get to sleep. Tea baths can be used during the same day as well. Of course, supplements can be added in, but if you are using teas make sure to tell your doctor that you're taking the herbal tea with the supplement you choose. You'll find that most

can be paired together, and there's always a
natural solution for your sleep problems.

www.ingramcontent.com/pod-product-compliance
Lightning Source LLC
Chambersburg PA
CBHW061034050726
47592CB00004B/1443